Mind Shift

Transform Your Thinking and Achieve Success

Mark West

Contents

Executive summary

This book provides a comprehensive guide to personal growth and achievement, focusing on practical strategies and actionable steps to help you transform your life. Each chapter explores a critical aspect of personal development, from setting clear goals and developing a growth mindset to embracing failure and cultivating positive habits.

Starting with the importance of goal-setting, the book shows you how to define specific, measurable, and achievable goals, breaking them down into manageable steps and creating a consistent action plan. It then delves into the role of reflection and adjustment, teaching you how to evaluate your progress, learn from setbacks, and refine your approach to stay on course.

The book emphasises the significance of self-care, mental well-being, and building strong relationships, showing how these areas are essential for long-term success. You'll also learn how to stay motivated, overcome plateaus, and take consistent action, no matter the obstacles that arise.

With a focus on creating habits that serve your goals, maintaining accountability, and cultivating resilience, the book equips you with the tools and mindset to pursue your dreams with purpose and determination. Through regular reflection, celebration of progress, and continuous learning, you will develop the clarity, confidence, and perseverance needed to achieve your full potential.

This book is an invitation to take control of your life, reflect on your values, and take consistent, intentional steps toward a more fulfilling and successful future. Whether you're looking to improve your career, personal life, or overall well-being, the principles in this book will guide you toward sustained growth and success.

Understanding the Foundation

Chapter 1: Identifying Your Goals

Introduction

Many of us go through life driven by routines and responsibilities, often without clearly defining what we truly want to achieve. Setting goals isn't just a motivational technique; it's the foundation upon which we build a purposeful life. When you identify and articulate your goals, you're setting a course to make your life more meaningful and directed.

Why Goal-Setting Matters

At its core, goal-setting is about clarity. It's about understanding the 'why' behind our actions and decisions. When we don't have goals, it's easy to become distracted by short-term desires or feel unmotivated. Goals give us a target, and with that target, we can measure our progress and push ourselves to achieve more than we might have believed possible.

Setting goals also impacts how we view challenges. When there's a meaningful aim in sight, obstacles become part of the journey rather than reasons to give up. You're not just "going through the motions"; you're actively pursuing a dream.

Step 1: Dream Big and Imagine Possibilities

To identify your goals, start by allowing yourself to dream. Here's a simple exercise: grab a piece of paper and divide it into four sections:

1. **Personal Life**: Think about your relationships, hobbies, and well-being.

2. **Career or Professional Goals**: Consider your job, business aspirations, or educational achievements.
3. **Financial Goals**: What do you want your financial future to look like?
4. **Contribution to Society**: Think about how you want to impact the world around you.

Write down as many ideas as possible in each section. This process isn't about limitation or perfection; it's about envisioning what you'd ideally want if anything were possible.

Step 2: Narrow Down and Prioritise

Once you've identified potential goals, it's time to refine them. Look at your list and pick the top two or three goals in each category that resonate with you the most. A good way to determine which goals hold the most value is to ask yourself why each one is important to you.

Asking "why" is crucial because it helps you connect emotionally with your goals. For example, if you've listed "getting fit," dig deeper and ask why. Is it to improve your health, to feel more confident, or to have more energy for loved ones? The deeper your connection to the goal, the more likely you are to commit to it.

Step 3: Make Your Goals Specific and Measurable

One reason people struggle with achieving goals is because they are too vague. Goals should be clear and measurable. For example, rather than setting a goal to "be healthier," try making it specific: "I want to lose 10 pounds in the next three months by exercising three times a week and eating balanced meals."

Using the SMART framework is a great way to make goals effective:

- **Specific**: What exactly do you want to achieve?

- **Measurable**: How will you know when you've achieved it?
- **Achievable**: Is this goal within your reach?
- **Relevant**: Does this goal matter to your life and values?
- **Time-Bound**: What is the deadline for achieving this goal?

Step 4: Break Down Goals into Actionable Steps

Big goals can sometimes feel overwhelming. Breaking them down into smaller, actionable steps helps make the journey more manageable. For instance, if your goal is to write a book, your first step might be to draft an outline, then to write a certain number of words each day.

Create a list of milestones for each goal. These should be smaller achievements that lead up to the bigger goal. Not only does this approach make the process less intimidating, but it also allows you to celebrate progress along the way, keeping you motivated.

Step 5: Create a Visual Representation of Your Goals

Our minds respond well to visuals, so creating a vision board or a list that you can look at daily can reinforce your commitment to your goals. Include images, words, and anything that reminds you of why you set these goals in the first place. Place it somewhere visible to keep your aspirations front and centre.

Step 6: Hold Yourself Accountable

One of the keys to success is accountability. Find a friend, family member, or colleague who will support you. Check in with them regularly to share your progress. Alternatively, consider keeping a journal where you track your steps toward each goal, noting both successes and setbacks.

Accountability helps you stay honest with yourself. When you know someone else is tracking your journey, you're more likely to stick to your commitments.

Step 7: Re-evaluate and Adjust as Needed

Life changes, and so will your goals. Periodically reviewing your goals and progress is essential. Maybe some goals will no longer feel relevant, or new priorities will emerge. Give yourself the flexibility to adjust without feeling discouraged. Progress is rarely a straight line; it's about moving in the right direction, even if the path changes.

Reflection and Encouragement

At this point, you've likely pinpointed a few goals that feel meaningful. Remember, the journey you're beginning is just as important as the destination. Each small step brings you closer to a more fulfilling life. As you move forward, hold onto the vision you've created here in this chapter, and trust in your ability to make it a reality.

Practical Steps for Transformation

Chapter 2: Understanding Limiting Beliefs

Introduction

Setting goals is an essential first step, but many people struggle to move forward due to hidden barriers rooted in their own minds. These barriers, often called *limiting beliefs*, are subconscious ideas that restrict what we believe we can achieve. This chapter will guide you through understanding, identifying, and challenging these beliefs, freeing you to pursue your goals without self-imposed limitations.

What Are Limiting Beliefs?

A limiting belief is any thought or perception that holds you back from reaching your potential. These beliefs often stem from past experiences, societal norms, or comments from influential people in our lives. For example, if you were told as a child that you weren't "clever enough," that idea can take root in your mind, impacting your confidence even decades later.

Common limiting beliefs sound like:

- "I'm not good enough to succeed in this."
- "I don't deserve happiness."
- "I'll probably fail, so why even try?"
- "People like me can't achieve things like that."

These thoughts can be so ingrained that they feel like facts, even though they are not. Limiting beliefs often operate quietly in the background, influencing your actions and decisions without you even realising it.

The Power of Identifying Limiting Beliefs

To overcome limiting beliefs, you must first bring them to light. This requires self-reflection and a willingness to question long-held assumptions about yourself. Identifying your limiting beliefs is like locating the root of a weed; once you uncover the root, you can begin to pull it out and make space for new, healthier beliefs.

Step 1: Recognise Negative Self-Talk

One of the clearest indicators of a limiting belief is negative self-talk. Pay attention to how you speak to yourself, especially when facing challenges or considering new goals. Do you catch yourself thinking, "I'm not capable" or "This will never work"? Negative self-talk is often a direct reflection of the beliefs you hold.

Exercise:

- For one week, keep a journal of your self-talk. Each time you catch yourself thinking negatively about your abilities or goals, write it down.
- At the end of the week, review your entries. Look for patterns or repeated phrases—these are likely tied to limiting beliefs.

Step 2: Identify the Source of Your Limiting Beliefs

After you've recognised these beliefs, try to trace them back to their origin. Limiting beliefs often stem from specific past experiences or the influence of authority figures, such as parents, teachers, or peers. Ask yourself, "When did I start believing this?" and "Who influenced me to think this way?"

Understanding the source can help you separate past experiences from your current reality. For instance, if you have a limiting belief about money, it might stem from growing up in a financially unstable household. Recognising this link helps you see that the belief was shaped by circumstances that no longer apply.

Step 3: Question the Validity of Each Belief

Once you've identified a limiting belief, challenge its accuracy. Just because you believe something doesn't make it true. Often, these beliefs crumble under scrutiny.

Here are some questions to help challenge your limiting beliefs:

- "Is there evidence that contradicts this belief?"
- "Have I ever succeeded in a similar situation despite this belief?"
- "Would I say this about someone else in my position?"
- "What's the worst that could happen if I attempted to disprove this belief?"

Exercise:

- Take one limiting belief and write it down at the top of a page.
- Below it, write down any evidence you can find that disproves it. This could include past successes, compliments from others, or personal strengths that counter the belief.

Step 4: Replace Limiting Beliefs with Empowering Beliefs

Challenging your beliefs is the first step; replacing them with positive, empowering beliefs is the next. Empowering beliefs are affirmations or thoughts that support your goals and enhance your confidence. For example, if your limiting belief is "I'm not clever enough to start my own business," an empowering belief could be "I have the skills and dedication needed to succeed."

Creating new beliefs requires repetition. Each time you catch yourself falling back into negative self-talk, replace it with an empowering belief. Over time, these positive thoughts will become second nature.

Examples of empowering beliefs:

- "I am capable of learning and growing."
- "I deserve success and happiness."
- "Every effort I make brings me closer to my goals."

Step 5: Take Small, Confidence-Building Actions

One of the most effective ways to solidify a new belief is by taking actions that support it. Each small step reinforces your confidence and proves to your mind that the limiting belief isn't true.

For instance, if your limiting belief is that you're not good at public speaking, set a goal to speak up at a small meeting or join a group where you can practise speaking in front of others. These small actions serve as evidence that your new empowering belief is accurate.

Exercise:

- Write down one small, achievable action that aligns with an empowering belief.
- Take this action within the next week, and reflect on how it makes you feel. Document the experience to reinforce your progress.

Step 6: Surround Yourself with Positive Influences

Our beliefs are often influenced by the people around us. Surrounding yourself with supportive, positive individuals can help reinforce your empowering beliefs. Seek out mentors, friends, or communities that encourage growth and believe in your potential.

If you find yourself surrounded by people who reinforce negative beliefs, try limiting your exposure to them or seek support groups, online communities, or local meetups where positivity and personal growth are emphasised.

Moving Forward with New Beliefs

Rewriting limiting beliefs is not a one-time process; it's an ongoing journey. Overcoming these beliefs requires patience, but each small shift makes a significant difference. Every time you challenge a negative thought or take a step outside your comfort zone, you're breaking down the barriers that once held you back.

As you continue through this book, remind yourself of the empowering beliefs you're building. Keep reinforcing them, and you'll soon notice that the goals you set in Chapter 1 feel more achievable. With a stronger, more positive mindset, you're now equipped to face life's challenges with confidence.

Chapter 3: Developing a Growth Mindset

Introduction

In our pursuit of personal goals and fulfilment, the way we perceive challenges, setbacks, and our own abilities can make all the difference. A *growth mindset* is the belief that our abilities and intelligence can be developed with effort, learning, and perseverance. In contrast, a *fixed mindset* is the belief that these qualities are static and unchangeable. This chapter will guide you in adopting a growth mindset, allowing you to approach life with resilience and curiosity.

What is a Growth Mindset?

Psychologist Dr Carol Dweck, who pioneered the concept of the growth mindset, discovered that people with this mindset view challenges as opportunities to learn and grow. They believe that effort and perseverance can lead to improvement and success. Conversely, people with a fixed mindset avoid challenges for fear of failure, believing that their abilities are set in stone.

A growth mindset encourages you to see effort as a path to mastery rather than a sign of inadequacy. Instead of saying, "I can't do this," you begin to think, "I can't do this *yet*." This single word, "yet," transforms your mindset, reminding you that with time and practice, your abilities can develop.

Recognising Fixed Mindset Thinking

Cultivating a growth mindset begins with identifying and challenging fixed mindset thinking. Fixed mindset thoughts often sound like:

- "I'm just not good at this."
- "I'll never be as talented as others."
- "If I fail, it means I'm not capable."

- "I should stick to what I'm naturally good at."

Exercise:

- Spend a week tracking moments when you feel resistant to trying something new, when you fear failure, or when you criticise your abilities.
- Write these thoughts down and label them as "fixed mindset" thoughts. This practice will help you recognise patterns and realise how often a fixed mindset holds you back.

Step 1: Embrace Challenges as Opportunities

The first step to developing a growth mindset is to start viewing challenges as chances to learn. Instead of avoiding difficult tasks, actively seek out challenges that will push you out of your comfort zone.

Every challenge you encounter offers an opportunity to strengthen your skills and learn something new. Whether it's tackling a complex project at work, learning a new skill, or addressing a personal fear, approaching these challenges with an open mind builds resilience and adaptability.

Exercise:

- Choose one challenging task you've been avoiding, and set a plan to tackle it this week. Write down what you hope to learn or gain from the experience, even if it doesn't go perfectly.

Step 2: Value Effort Over Talent

In a fixed mindset, people often view effort as something only required by those who lack natural talent. However, a growth mindset sees effort as the essential ingredient for growth. Research consistently shows that even those with natural talent benefit tremendously from putting in consistent effort.

Replace thoughts like, "I'm not naturally good at this" with "I can improve through practice." Emphasising effort means recognising that growth is a process, and every attempt, regardless of the outcome, brings you closer to your goal.

Step 3: Learn from Feedback

Feedback is essential for growth, but it can be difficult to hear, especially when it points out areas for improvement. People with a fixed mindset often avoid feedback, viewing it as a criticism of their abilities. In contrast, those with a growth mindset see feedback as a valuable tool to help them improve.

When you receive feedback, try to see it as an opportunity to learn rather than a judgement of your abilities. Look at the specific points raised, and consider how they could help you get closer to your goal. If the feedback isn't constructive, remember that it's a reflection on the situation, not a statement about your potential.

Exercise:

- Think about recent feedback you received, whether at work or in your personal life. Write down the points that were highlighted and consider one action you could take based on this feedback.

Step 4: View Failures as Steps Toward Success

In a growth mindset, failures are not final—they're steps on the path to success. Every time you "fail," you gain information about what doesn't work, bringing you closer to understanding what does. Instead of seeing setbacks as a sign of inadequacy, try to reframe them as valuable learning experiences.

Whenever you experience a setback, ask yourself, "What can I learn from this experience?" By focusing on the lessons rather than the loss, you'll build resilience and a willingness to try again.

Exercise:

- Reflect on a recent failure or setback. Write down three things you learnt from the experience and consider how you could apply those lessons in the future.

Step 5: Celebrate Progress, Not Just Results

A growth mindset emphasises progress over perfection. People often fall into the trap of only celebrating end results, but recognising progress—even if it's incremental—helps sustain motivation.

Each step you take towards your goal is a small victory worth celebrating. By valuing progress, you reinforce the belief that growth is an ongoing journey, not a final destination. This approach also makes long-term goals feel more achievable, as you're focused on the next step rather than the entire journey.

Exercise:

- Choose a goal you're working on and make a list of the small steps you've taken towards achieving it. Each time you complete another step, take a moment to acknowledge your progress.

Surround Yourself with a Growth-Minded Environment

Your environment plays a huge role in shaping your mindset. Surround yourself with people who believe in growth and improvement and who encourage you to strive for your best. Having friends, mentors, or colleagues who model a growth mindset can inspire you to adopt the same attitude.

If you're in an environment where a fixed mindset dominates, seek out communities—whether online or offline—that prioritise learning, growth, and positive reinforcement. Finding people who share a growth mindset will strengthen your resolve and make your journey easier.

Moving Forward with a Growth Mindset

Developing a growth mindset is an ongoing process. As you move forward, continue to challenge yourself, seek out opportunities to learn, and reflect on your progress. Remember, a growth mindset is about believing in your capacity to grow and improve.

By embracing this mindset, you're empowering yourself to face challenges head-on, view failures as stepping stones, and persist when things get tough. As you cultivate a growth mindset, you'll find that you're more resilient, adaptable, and ready to make the most of your potential.

Chapter 4: Developing a Growth Mindset

Introduction

In our pursuit of personal goals and fulfilment, the way we perceive
challenges, setbacks, and our own abilities can make all the difference.
A *growth mindset* is the belief that our abilities and intelligence can be
developed with effort, learning, and perseverance. In contrast, a *fixed
mindset* is the belief that these qualities are static and unchangeable.
This chapter will guide you in adopting a growth mindset, allowing you
to approach life with resilience and curiosity.

What is a Growth Mindset?

Psychologist Dr Carol Dweck, who pioneered the concept of the growth
mindset, discovered that people with this mindset view challenges as
opportunities to learn and grow. They believe that effort and
perseverance can lead to improvement and success. Conversely, people
with a fixed mindset avoid challenges for fear of failure, believing that
their abilities are set in stone.

A growth mindset encourages you to see effort as a path to mastery
rather than a sign of inadequacy. Instead of saying, "I can't do this,"
you begin to think, "I can't do this *yet*." This single word, "yet,"
transforms your mindset, reminding you that with time and practice,
your abilities can develop.

Recognising Fixed Mindset Thinking

Cultivating a growth mindset begins with identifying and challenging
fixed mindset thinking. Fixed mindset thoughts often sound like:

- "I'm just not good at this."
- "I'll never be as talented as others."
- "If I fail, it means I'm not capable."

- "I should stick to what I'm naturally good at."

Exercise:

- Spend a week tracking moments when you feel resistant to trying something new, when you fear failure, or when you criticise your abilities.
- Write these thoughts down and label them as "fixed mindset" thoughts. This practice will help you recognise patterns and realise how often a fixed mindset holds you back.

Step 1: Embrace Challenges as Opportunities

The first step to developing a growth mindset is to start viewing challenges as chances to learn. Instead of avoiding difficult tasks, actively seek out challenges that will push you out of your comfort zone.

Every challenge you encounter offers an opportunity to strengthen your skills and learn something new. Whether it's tackling a complex project at work, learning a new skill, or addressing a personal fear, approaching these challenges with an open mind builds resilience and adaptability.

Exercise:

- Choose one challenging task you've been avoiding, and set a plan to tackle it this week. Write down what you hope to learn or gain from the experience, even if it doesn't go perfectly.

Step 2: Value Effort Over Talent

In a fixed mindset, people often view effort as something only required by those who lack natural talent. However, a growth mindset sees effort as the essential ingredient for growth. Research consistently shows that even those with natural talent benefit tremendously from putting in consistent effort.

Replace thoughts like, "I'm not naturally good at this" with "I can improve through practice." Emphasising effort means recognising that growth is a process, and every attempt, regardless of the outcome, brings you closer to your goal.

Step 3: Learn from Feedback

Feedback is essential for growth, but it can be difficult to hear, especially when it points out areas for improvement. People with a fixed mindset often avoid feedback, viewing it as a criticism of their abilities. In contrast, those with a growth mindset see feedback as a valuable tool to help them improve.

When you receive feedback, try to see it as an opportunity to learn rather than a judgement of your abilities. Look at the specific points raised, and consider how they could help you get closer to your goal. If the feedback isn't constructive, remember that it's a reflection on the situation, not a statement about your potential.

Exercise:

- Think about recent feedback you received, whether at work or in your personal life. Write down the points that were highlighted and consider one action you could take based on this feedback.

Step 4: View Failures as Steps Toward Success

In a growth mindset, failures are not final—they're steps on the path to success. Every time you "fail," you gain information about what doesn't work, bringing you closer to understanding what does. Instead of seeing setbacks as a sign of inadequacy, try to reframe them as valuable learning experiences.

Whenever you experience a setback, ask yourself, "What can I learn from this experience?" By focusing on the lessons rather than the loss, you'll build resilience and a willingness to try again.

Exercise:

- Reflect on a recent failure or setback. Write down three things you learnt from the experience and consider how you could apply those lessons in the future.

Step 5: Celebrate Progress, Not Just Results

A growth mindset emphasises progress over perfection. People often fall into the trap of only celebrating end results, but recognising progress—even if it's incremental—helps sustain motivation.

Each step you take towards your goal is a small victory worth celebrating. By valuing progress, you reinforce the belief that growth is an ongoing journey, not a final destination. This approach also makes long-term goals feel more achievable, as you're focused on the next step rather than the entire journey.

Exercise:

- Choose a goal you're working on and make a list of the small steps you've taken towards achieving it. Each time you complete another step, take a moment to acknowledge your progress.

Surround Yourself with a Growth-Minded Environment

Your environment plays a huge role in shaping your mindset. Surround yourself with people who believe in growth and improvement and who encourage you to strive for your best. Having friends, mentors, or colleagues who model a growth mindset can inspire you to adopt the same attitude.

If you're in an environment where a fixed mindset dominates, seek out communities—whether online or offline—that prioritise learning, growth, and positive reinforcement. Finding people who share a growth mindset will strengthen your resolve and make your journey easier.

Moving Forward with a Growth Mindset

Developing a growth mindset is an ongoing process. As you move forward, continue to challenge yourself, seek out opportunities to learn, and reflect on your progress. Remember, a growth mindset is about believing in your capacity to grow and improve.

By embracing this mindset, you're empowering yourself to face challenges head-on, view failures as stepping stones, and persist when things get tough. As you cultivate a growth mindset, you'll find that you're more resilient, adaptable, and ready to make the most of your potential.

Chapter 5: Embracing Failure as a Learning Tool

Introduction

Failure is often viewed as something to be avoided at all costs. We fear the disappointment, the embarrassment, and the sense of inadequacy that can come with failing. However, failure is an essential part of growth and learning. When we embrace failure as a valuable learning tool, it becomes a stepping stone towards success rather than a roadblock. This chapter will help you shift your perspective on failure and harness its potential to fuel your progress.

Why Failure Matters

At first glance, failure may seem like a setback or an indication that we're not good enough. However, if you look closer, failure is simply feedback. It's a way of gaining insight into what isn't working, which ultimately helps guide you towards what will work. Every successful person has encountered failure, often repeatedly. The difference lies in how they responded. Instead of giving up, they used those experiences to adapt and improve.

Embracing failure means acknowledging that it's a natural part of the journey, especially when you're pursuing meaningful goals or challenging yourself to grow.

Step 1: Redefine Failure

One of the first steps in embracing failure is to redefine what it means to fail. Failure doesn't mean that you're incapable or that you'll never succeed. It simply means that your current approach didn't yield the results you wanted. This distinction is crucial because it allows you to separate your self-worth from the outcome.

By viewing failure as a temporary result, you're opening the door to growth. Instead of saying, "I failed," try saying, "That approach didn't work. What can I do differently?" This small shift in language encourages you to think of failure as an opportunity to try new methods.

Exercise:

- Reflect on a time when you felt you had "failed." Write down what happened, but focus on the actions or circumstances rather than yourself as a person.
- Reframe this experience by writing a sentence that separates you from the outcome, such as, "This attempt didn't work, but I can learn from it."

Step 2: Analyse the Lessons in Every Setback

Each failure holds valuable lessons, but only if you're willing to analyse it honestly. When something doesn't go as planned, resist the urge to dwell on the disappointment. Instead, focus on what you can learn from the experience.

Ask yourself questions such as:

- "What specifically didn't work, and why?"
- "Is there something I could do differently next time?"
- "What did I learn about myself, my skills, or my approach?"

This analysis helps you gain clarity and direction. You may discover gaps in your knowledge, areas for improvement, or even external factors that influenced the outcome. Use this information to make adjustments and move forward with a stronger, more informed approach.

Exercise:

- Think of a recent setback. Write down three specific lessons
  you learnt from it. How can you apply these lessons in future
  attempts?

Step 3: Cultivate Resilience Through Repeated Attempts

One of the key traits shared by those who succeed is resilience.
Resilience is the ability to keep going in the face of adversity, and it's
something that develops each time you push through failure. When you
experience a setback, it's easy to feel discouraged or to lose motivation.
However, by viewing each attempt as part of the process, you're
training yourself to bounce back stronger.

With each failure, remind yourself that you're building resilience. The
more you persevere, the more equipped you'll be to face future
challenges with confidence. This doesn't mean ignoring the feelings
that come with failure, but rather acknowledging them and continuing
despite them.

Step 4: Celebrate Your Efforts, Not Just the Outcome

Our society tends to celebrate end results, which can lead us to feel that
anything less than success isn't worth acknowledging. However, the
effort you put into each attempt, regardless of the result, is a significant
achievement in itself. When you start to value your efforts rather than
only the outcome, you're reinforcing a growth mindset and fostering
self-encouragement.

Celebrating effort means recognising your commitment, determination,
and willingness to take risks. Each time you make an effort, you're
moving closer to your goal, even if the progress isn't immediately
visible.

Exercise:

- Think of an effort you made recently, even if it didn't yield the result you wanted. Write down what you're proud of in that attempt, focusing on the effort, skills, or courage it took.

Step 5: Embrace a Long-Term Perspective

When we face failure, it's natural to focus on the immediate disappointment. However, most worthwhile accomplishments require a long-term perspective. Progress is rarely linear; it's made up of ups and downs, small wins, and setbacks. By keeping a long-term view, you're less likely to be discouraged by short-term failures.

When you look back on your journey, you'll realise that each failure contributed to your growth, even if it didn't seem that way at the time. Embracing this perspective can help you appreciate the entire process rather than only the end result.

Exercise:

- Reflect on a goal you achieved in the past and consider any failures or setbacks you encountered along the way. How did those moments contribute to your overall success?

Letting Go of the Fear of Failure

The fear of failure can be paralysing, preventing us from taking risks or pursuing new opportunities. To let go of this fear, start by shifting your mindset. Remind yourself that failure is not a reflection of your worth but a natural part of learning and growth.

The more you experience failure and learn from it, the less you'll fear it. Failure loses its power when you realise it's simply a stepping stone. By facing this fear, you'll find that you're able to tackle bigger challenges and take on new opportunities with confidence.

Moving Forward with a Growth-Oriented Approach

Embracing failure as a learning tool is a transformative step towards achieving your goals. Each setback becomes an opportunity to grow, to refine your approach, and to build resilience. As you continue on your journey, remember that failure is simply part of the process. The path to success is rarely a straight line, but with each failure, you're learning, adapting, and getting closer to your ultimate goal.

With this growth-oriented approach, you're equipped to face challenges head-on, take risks, and pursue your aspirations with resilience and courage.

Chapter 6: Building Confidence Through Action

Introduction

Confidence is a powerful force that influences nearly every aspect of our lives, from personal relationships to career opportunities. While some people seem naturally confident, confidence isn't an inherent trait; it's something that can be developed through practice and experience. This chapter will explore how taking consistent, purposeful action can help you build and strengthen your confidence over time.

The Link Between Action and Confidence

One of the most effective ways to build confidence is by taking action. Every time you take a step towards your goals, even a small one, you're proving to yourself that you're capable. Confidence grows when we challenge ourselves and overcome obstacles, no matter how minor.

Confidence is often mistaken for the absence of fear, but true confidence involves recognising fear and moving forward regardless. Each action you take, despite any nerves or hesitation, reinforces your belief in your abilities.

Step 1: Start Small and Build Momentum

When it comes to building confidence, starting with small, manageable actions can make a huge difference. Trying to tackle a major challenge right away can be overwhelming, especially if you're already struggling with self-doubt. Instead, break your goal down into smaller, achievable steps. Each step you complete successfully adds to your confidence.

For instance, if your goal is to speak confidently in public, begin by practising in front of a mirror or with a small group of friends. As you get comfortable with each step, gradually increase the difficulty until you're ready to face the larger challenge.

Exercise:

- Write down a goal you'd like to achieve. Break it down into at least five small steps. Focus on completing one step at a time, celebrating each small success along the way.

Step 2: Focus on Preparation and Skill-Building

Confidence isn't just a mindset; it's also a result of preparation and skill. The more prepared you are, the more confident you'll feel. For example, if you're nervous about a job interview, taking the time to research the company, practice answering questions, and review your skills will help reduce anxiety and boost your self-assurance.

Developing your skills in areas where you feel less confident can also build your self-belief. Learning, practising, and improving in specific areas will reinforce your ability to handle challenges, which, in turn, strengthens your confidence.

Exercise:

- Think about an area where you lack confidence. Identify one or two skills you could improve to feel more prepared. Make a plan to start practising these skills over the coming weeks.

Step 3: Embrace a Growth Mindset and View Mistakes as Learning Opportunities

As we discussed in previous chapters, a growth mindset is the belief that your abilities can be developed through effort and learning. When it comes to confidence, a growth mindset is invaluable because it allows you to view mistakes as opportunities for growth rather than as failures.

Every time you make a mistake, remind yourself that it's part of the learning process. Instead of dwelling on what went wrong, focus on what you can do differently next time. This mindset enables you to keep moving forward, even after setbacks, which builds resilience and confidence.

Exercise:

- Reflect on a recent situation where you felt you made a mistake. Write down what happened and, instead of focusing on the negative, list three things you learnt from the experience. Think about how you can apply these lessons in future situations.

Step 4: Practise Positive Self-Talk and Visualisation

Self-talk, the inner dialogue we have with ourselves, has a significant impact on our confidence. Negative self-talk can undermine your confidence, while positive self-talk can empower you to take action. When you catch yourself thinking, "I can't do this" or "I'm not good enough," replace these thoughts with affirmations like "I am capable" or "I am learning and improving."

Visualisation is another powerful tool for building confidence. Imagine yourself successfully completing a task or achieving a goal. Picture the setting, the people around you, and your feelings of accomplishment. Visualising success can help reinforce your belief in your abilities and make you more likely to take action.

Exercise:

- Choose an upcoming situation where you'd like to feel more confident. Spend a few minutes each day visualising yourself succeeding in that situation. As you visualise, repeat a positive affirmation, such as "I am prepared and capable."

Step 5: Take Risks and Expand Your Comfort Zone

Confidence grows when you push yourself beyond your comfort zone. While it may feel safe to stick to familiar tasks, true growth requires taking risks. This doesn't mean taking unnecessary risks, but rather challenging yourself to try new things, even if they feel intimidating.

Each time you take a risk and step outside your comfort zone, you're proving to yourself that you can handle the unknown. Even if things don't go perfectly, the act of trying something new builds resilience and self-assurance.

Exercise:

- Identify one action that's slightly outside your comfort zone, whether it's speaking up in a meeting, trying a new skill, or attending a social event alone. Set a date to take this action within the next week, and reflect on how it made you feel afterwards.

Step 6: Surround Yourself with Supportive People

The people you surround yourself with play a huge role in shaping your confidence. Supportive friends, family members, or mentors can encourage you to pursue your goals, offer valuable feedback, and remind you of your strengths. On the other hand, negative or critical people can drain your confidence and reinforce self-doubt.

Seek out individuals who believe in your potential and want to see you succeed. Let their encouragement inspire you, and, whenever possible, avoid people who consistently undermine your confidence.

Exercise:

- Take a moment to reflect on the people in your life. Who are the ones that encourage you and make you feel confident? Consider reaching out to one of these individuals this week to discuss your goals and gain some positive reinforcement.

Moving Forward with Confidence

Building confidence is a gradual process that requires consistent action. Each small step, each new skill, and each supportive conversation contributes to a growing belief in your abilities. Confidence isn't about being fearless; it's about acknowledging your fears and taking action anyway.

As you continue through this book and your personal journey, keep challenging yourself to take steps—no matter how small—towards your goals. With each action, you're building a foundation of confidence that will support you in achieving your dreams.

Chapter 7: Time Management and Prioritisation

Introduction

Time is one of our most valuable resources, yet it often feels as though there's never enough of it. Effective time management isn't about squeezing as much as possible into each day; it's about making thoughtful choices that allow you to focus on what matters most. This chapter will provide practical strategies for managing your time effectively and prioritising tasks, so you can make steady progress towards your goals.

Why Time Management Matters

Good time management empowers you to take control of your life rather than letting your to-do list dictate your day. It reduces stress, boosts productivity, and ensures that you're dedicating time to the things that align with your values and goals. Without a strategy for managing time, it's easy to become overwhelmed, distracted, or even discouraged.

By managing your time effectively, you're also prioritising yourself and your goals. You're acknowledging that your time and energy are finite resources that should be spent on what truly matters.

Step 1: Identify Your Priorities

Before you can manage your time effectively, you need to clarify what's most important to you. Ask yourself: "What are the three or four things in my life that matter most right now?" These might include career, family, health, personal development, or specific goals you've set for yourself.

Once you've identified these priorities, use them as a guide for how you spend your time. When you're clear on what matters, it becomes easier to let go of tasks or commitments that don't align with these priorities.

Exercise:

- Make a list of your top priorities. Next to each priority, write down a few actions that would help you progress in that area. Keep this list visible as a reminder of where to focus your time and energy.

Step 2: Break Down Goals into Manageable Tasks

Big goals can feel overwhelming, making it difficult to know where to start. Breaking them down into smaller, manageable tasks helps make the process more achievable and less intimidating. When each step is clearly defined, it's easier to take action without feeling overwhelmed.

For example, if your goal is to write a book, break it down into tasks like "brainstorm chapter ideas," "write an outline," and "write 500 words each day." Each of these smaller tasks brings you closer to completing the larger goal.

Exercise:

- Choose one of your major goals and break it down into smaller tasks. Write these tasks down in a to-do list format, and aim to complete one or two of them each week.

Step 3: Use Time-Blocking to Structure Your Day

Time-blocking is a powerful technique for managing your day. It involves dividing your day into blocks of time, with each block dedicated to a specific task or activity. This approach helps you focus on one task at a time, making you more productive and reducing the likelihood of distractions.

Start by blocking out time for your most important tasks first. Then allocate blocks for other activities, including breaks and personal time. Stick to your time blocks as closely as possible, but be flexible if something urgent comes up.

Exercise:

- Choose a day this week to practise time-blocking. Plan your day in advance, allocating specific blocks for different tasks. After the day is over, reflect on how it affected your productivity and focus.

Step 4: Learn to Say "No" and Protect Your Time

One of the biggest challenges in time management is saying "no" to tasks, invitations, or commitments that don't align with your priorities. Many of us feel compelled to say "yes" out of politeness, obligation, or fear of missing out, but overcommitting can quickly lead to burnout and prevent you from focusing on what matters.

When faced with a new request or opportunity, take a moment to consider whether it aligns with your goals. If it doesn't, give yourself permission to decline. Politely but firmly saying "no" frees up your time for activities that contribute to your growth and well-being.

Exercise:

- Think about any commitments you've taken on recently that may not align with your priorities. Identify one that you could let go of or reduce. Practise saying "no" in a way that feels comfortable to you.

Step 5: Minimise Distractions and Maintain Focus

In today's digital world, distractions are everywhere—from constant notifications to the lure of social media. Minimising distractions is crucial for effective time management, as it allows you to focus on tasks without being pulled in multiple directions.

Consider setting specific times to check emails or social media, rather than letting them interrupt your work throughout the day. If necessary, use tools or apps that block certain sites or silence notifications during work hours. Creating a distraction-free environment allows you to work more efficiently, freeing up time for other priorities.

Exercise:

- Identify your top three distractions. Write down a strategy to minimise each one. For example, you might turn off phone notifications, use a productivity app, or create a designated workspace.

Step 6: Regularly Review and Adjust Your Schedule

Life is constantly changing, and so are our priorities. Regularly reviewing your schedule and adjusting it as needed ensures that your time management remains aligned with your current goals. Take a few minutes each week to assess what went well, what didn't, and where adjustments might be needed.

This weekly review process can help you spot time-wasting activities, refine your approach, and make sure that you're always moving closer to your goals.

Exercise:

- Set aside 15 minutes at the end of each week to review your schedule. Reflect on how you spent your time, celebrate any progress you made, and note any areas where you'd like to improve.

Embracing a Balanced Approach to Time Management

Effective time management isn't about being constantly busy; it's about working smarter and focusing on what truly matters. By identifying your priorities, breaking down tasks, minimising distractions, and making room for flexibility, you're setting yourself up for a balanced, fulfilling life.

Time is one of the few resources we can never get back, so use it wisely. Remember that how you spend your time is ultimately how you're spending your life. With thoughtful planning and clear priorities, you'll find that you're able to make steady progress towards your goals while still enjoying the present.

Practical Steps for Transformation

Chapter 8: Building Positive Habits

Introduction

Habits shape our lives more than we often realise. The small decisions we make daily can either move us closer to our goals or keep us stuck in patterns that don't serve us. Building positive habits is one of the most powerful ways to create lasting change and achieve success. This chapter will explore how to build habits that support your goals and lead to long-term personal growth.

Why Habits Matter

Habits are the small actions we repeat regularly, often without thinking. Whether we realise it or not, they play a significant role in determining the quality of our lives. Positive habits, such as exercising regularly, eating healthily, or practising gratitude, can improve our physical and mental well-being, increase productivity, and help us achieve our long-term goals.

On the other hand, negative habits, like procrastination, poor sleep, or unhealthy eating, can undermine our progress. Since habits are formed through repetition, they can either work for us or against us. The key is to focus on building the right habits and letting go of those that no longer serve us.

Step 1: Start Small and Build Gradually

When it comes to building new habits, starting small is key. Trying to overhaul your entire life all at once can lead to burnout and frustration. Instead, choose one habit to focus on and begin with a small, manageable action.

For example, if your goal is to exercise more, start by committing to 10 minutes a day rather than an hour. Once this small habit is firmly established, you can gradually increase the time or intensity. Small steps make the process feel more achievable, and the progress you make will motivate you to continue.

Exercise:

- Choose one habit you'd like to develop. Break it down into a tiny, manageable step that you can commit to each day. For example, if you want to read more, start by reading just five pages a day.

Step 2: Create a Consistent Routine

Consistency is one of the most important factors in habit formation. The more consistently you perform a habit, the more it becomes ingrained in your routine. To build consistency, try to do your habit at the same time each day, ideally as part of an existing routine.

For example, if you want to meditate, consider doing it right after you wake up or just before bed. Pairing a new habit with an existing one—such as having a cup of tea after your morning jog—makes it easier to remember and integrate into your day.

Exercise:

- Identify a daily routine or trigger that you can use to prompt your new habit. For example, you might choose to exercise after your morning coffee or write in a journal before you go to bed. Make this pairing consistent every day.

Step 3: Make Your Habit Enjoyable

The more enjoyable a habit is, the more likely you are to stick with it. If you find yourself dreading a new habit, it will be much harder to maintain. Look for ways to make the habit enjoyable or rewarding.

For instance, if you're trying to eat more vegetables, experiment with different recipes or find a way to make healthy eating fun. If you want to exercise more, choose an activity that you genuinely enjoy, such as dancing, swimming, or walking in nature.

Adding an element of enjoyment not only makes the habit easier to stick to, but it also makes it something you look forward to. This positive reinforcement increases the likelihood that you'll continue with it long-term.

Exercise:

- Think about one new habit you're working on. Brainstorm ways to make it more enjoyable or rewarding. If your goal is to exercise, consider trying different activities until you find one that you genuinely love.

Step 4: Track Your Progress and Celebrate Small Wins

Tracking your progress is a great way to stay motivated and build momentum. By keeping track of your habits, you can see how far you've come, which can be incredibly motivating. Use a habit tracker or a simple journal to note your progress each day.

In addition to tracking, celebrate your small wins. Every time you complete your habit, give yourself a mental or physical reward. This could be as simple as acknowledging your achievement or treating yourself to something you enjoy. Celebrating your progress helps reinforce the habit and makes it feel rewarding.

Exercise:

- Create a habit tracker for the habit you're focusing on. Each day that you complete the habit, mark it on your tracker. At the end of the week, reward yourself with something small, such as a relaxing bath or a favourite treat.

Step 5: Be Patient and Allow for Setbacks

Habits take time to form, and it's normal to face setbacks along the way. It's important not to get discouraged if you miss a day or struggle to stay consistent. The key is to get back on track as soon as possible. Remember, building habits is a long-term process, and one mistake doesn't mean failure.

Instead of being harsh with yourself, practise self-compassion. Understand that setbacks are part of the learning process and are opportunities for growth. The more you can move past them without losing confidence, the easier it will be to maintain your habits.

Exercise:

- Reflect on a past setback where you struggled to keep up with a habit. Write down how you handled it and what you could do differently next time to get back on track. Practising patience and self-compassion is essential for building lasting habits.

Step 6: Use the Power of Habit Stacking

Habit stacking is a technique where you take an existing habit and "stack" a new habit on top of it. This method works well because it links a new behaviour with something you already do consistently.

For example, if you already brush your teeth every morning, you can stack a new habit, such as doing a short stretching routine, immediately after brushing your teeth. The existing habit acts as a trigger, making it easier to remember and incorporate the new habit.

Exercise:

- Think of one of your current habits that you already do consistently (e.g., drinking coffee, getting ready for work). Choose a small habit that you'd like to start and add it to the routine you already have.

Moving Forward with Consistent Habits

Building positive habits is a gradual process that takes time, patience, and effort. However, with consistent practice and a thoughtful approach, habits can become an integral part of your life. The key is to focus on small, manageable steps, make the habit enjoyable, and celebrate your progress along the way.

By building positive habits, you're setting yourself up for success in all areas of your life. As these habits become ingrained in your routine, you'll begin to see the long-term results they can bring, helping you achieve your goals and live a more fulfilling life.

Chapter 9: Practising Self-Care and Mental Well-being

Introduction

In our fast-paced world, it's easy to neglect our mental and physical well-being in the rush to meet deadlines, fulfil responsibilities, and meet others' expectations. However, self-care is not just a luxury or a once-in-a-while indulgence—it's an essential practice that nurtures your health, resilience, and overall happiness. In this chapter, we will explore the importance of self-care, practical steps to incorporate it into your life, and ways to prioritise mental well-being.

Why Self-Care Matters

Self-care refers to the activities and practices we engage in to promote our own physical, mental, and emotional health. While it's often associated with pampering or relaxation, true self-care goes beyond indulgence. It's about recognising your own needs, setting boundaries, and prioritising your well-being in order to lead a balanced and fulfilling life.

When we neglect self-care, stress and burnout can take a toll on both our body and mind. Practising self-care helps to reduce stress, enhance your mood, improve productivity, and create a sense of balance. It ensures that you're able to show up as your best self for others and maintain your own well-being.

Step 1: Prioritise Rest and Sleep

One of the cornerstones of self-care is proper rest. Sleep is vital for both your physical and mental health, and yet it's often one of the first things we sacrifice in our busy lives. Poor sleep can lead to irritability, a lack of focus, and a weakened immune system. In the long term, chronic sleep deprivation can contribute to more serious health issues, such as anxiety, depression, and heart disease.

To prioritise sleep, establish a consistent bedtime routine that promotes relaxation. This could include winding down without screens, having a warm bath, or practising mindfulness. Aim for 7-9 hours of sleep each night and create a sleep-friendly environment by keeping your room cool, dark, and quiet.

Exercise:

- Reflect on your current sleep habits. Are there any patterns or habits that are negatively affecting your sleep? Commit to one change that could help improve the quality of your rest—for example, limiting screen time before bed or establishing a calming pre-sleep routine.

Step 2: Nourish Your Body with Healthy Food

Your physical health is closely linked to your mental well-being. The foods you eat directly impact your mood, energy levels, and cognitive function. Eating a balanced, nutritious diet can help you feel more energised, improve concentration, and stabilise your emotions.

Rather than focusing on restrictive diets, aim to nourish your body with a variety of whole foods—vegetables, fruits, lean proteins, whole grains, and healthy fats. Drinking plenty of water and limiting processed foods can also support your overall well-being.

Exercise:

- Take note of your current eating habits. Are there any areas where you could improve your diet, such as adding more vegetables or drinking more water? Try incorporating one healthy change into your meals this week and observe how it affects your mood and energy.

Step 3: Move Your Body Regularly

Exercise is another essential component of self-care. Regular physical activity is not only good for your body but also boosts mental health. Exercise releases endorphins, which are natural mood boosters, and can help alleviate symptoms of anxiety and depression.

You don't need to commit to intense workouts; even a short daily walk, yoga, or stretching can make a significant difference. The key is to find an activity that you enjoy and can incorporate into your routine. This will make it easier to stick with and reap the benefits over time.

Exercise:

- Choose an activity you enjoy and commit to doing it for 20-30 minutes at least three times a week. Whether it's walking, dancing, or cycling, find something that feels good to you and helps you de-stress.

Step 4: Set Boundaries to Protect Your Energy

One of the most important aspects of self-care is setting boundaries. Often, we say "yes" to others at the expense of our own needs, leading to burnout and resentment. Learning to say "no" when necessary is a vital skill for preserving your time, energy, and mental health.

Boundaries help protect your well-being by ensuring that you don't overcommit yourself or allow others to drain your emotional resources. Setting clear boundaries with work, family, and social obligations helps you create space for self-care and personal time.

Exercise:

- Identify one area in your life where you need to set stronger boundaries. It could be with work, social events, or personal relationships. Practice saying "no" or politely setting limits to protect your energy and well-being.

Step 5: Foster Positive Relationships and Social Connections

Our mental well-being is deeply influenced by our relationships. Positive, supportive relationships can boost your mood, enhance your sense of belonging, and provide emotional support when needed. On the other hand, toxic or draining relationships can contribute to stress and anxiety.

It's important to surround yourself with people who uplift and encourage you. This doesn't mean cutting out everyone who may be difficult, but rather prioritising relationships that are nurturing and fulfilling. Additionally, make time for social connections, whether it's spending time with loved ones or engaging in community activities.

Exercise:

- Reflect on the relationships in your life. Are there any people who consistently bring you joy and support? Make a plan to connect with one of these individuals this week—whether in person, over the phone, or through a message.

Step 6: Practise Mindfulness and Stress Management

Mindfulness is a powerful tool for managing stress and maintaining mental clarity. By practising mindfulness, you can learn to stay present in the moment rather than getting caught up in worries about the past or future. Mindfulness helps to calm the mind, reduce stress, and improve emotional regulation.

You can practise mindfulness through meditation, breathing exercises, or simply paying attention to your thoughts and sensations throughout the day. Even a few minutes of mindful breathing can help centre your mind and reduce feelings of overwhelm.

Exercise:

- Try a simple mindfulness exercise: sit quietly for five minutes, close your eyes, and focus on your breath. Notice how the air feels as you inhale and exhale. If your mind wanders, gently bring your attention back to your breath. Practise this daily for a week and notice any changes in your stress levels.

Step 7: Engage in Activities That Bring You Joy

In the midst of daily responsibilities, it's easy to forget the activities that bring us joy. Whether it's a hobby, creative pursuit, or simply spending time in nature, engaging in activities you love is an important part of self-care.

These activities provide a sense of fulfilment and relaxation, helping to recharge your mental and emotional batteries. Make time for activities that make you feel alive, whether that's reading, painting, gardening, or listening to music.

Exercise:

- Identify one activity that brings you joy but that you've been neglecting. Schedule time for it in your week, whether it's an hour on the weekend or a few minutes each day.

Moving Forward with Self-Care

Self-care is not a one-off task; it's a lifelong practice that requires attention, awareness, and intention. By making self-care a priority, you are nurturing your well-being and building resilience to face life's challenges. Incorporating small, meaningful practices into your daily routine can have a profound impact on your mental health, energy levels, and overall quality of life.

Remember, self-care is not selfish—it's essential. By taking care of yourself, you ensure that you can show up as your best self for others and that you are equipped to live a fulfilling, balanced life.

Chapter 10: Cultivating Relationships and Support Systems

Introduction

Our relationships with others are fundamental to our emotional well-being and overall happiness. Whether it's family, friends, colleagues, or mentors, the people we surround ourselves with have a significant impact on our lives. Cultivating positive relationships and building a strong support system can provide us with the encouragement, advice, and emotional support we need to thrive. This chapter explores the importance of relationships and how to build a supportive network that enhances your personal and professional growth.

Why Relationships Matter

Healthy, supportive relationships contribute to our mental, emotional, and even physical well-being. Studies have shown that people with strong social connections are more resilient to stress, experience less anxiety and depression, and live longer, healthier lives. On the other hand, isolation and toxic relationships can have the opposite effect, leading to feelings of loneliness, stress, and poor mental health.

Building and maintaining positive relationships fosters a sense of belonging and connection, which is vital for our happiness and success. In both our personal and professional lives, relationships offer opportunities for growth, learning, and emotional support.

Step 1: Build Meaningful Connections

The first step in cultivating a strong support system is to build meaningful relationships. This doesn't mean having a large number of acquaintances, but rather focusing on the quality of your connections. Meaningful relationships are based on mutual respect, trust, and understanding.

Take the time to genuinely get to know others and show interest in their lives. Ask questions, listen actively, and be open to forming deeper connections. Whether it's a colleague, neighbour, or someone you meet through a shared interest, make an effort to nurture relationships that offer support and fulfilment.

Exercise:

- Identify one person in your life with whom you would like to build a stronger connection. Reach out to them with the intention of deepening your relationship—perhaps by inviting them for a coffee or having a more meaningful conversation.

Step 2: Foster Emotional Intelligence

Emotional intelligence (EI) is the ability to recognise, understand, and manage your emotions, as well as the emotions of others. High emotional intelligence allows you to navigate social situations with empathy and understanding, making it easier to build and maintain strong relationships.

To cultivate emotional intelligence, practise active listening, acknowledge the feelings of others, and manage your own emotions effectively. When you understand and manage emotions—both yours and others'—you can respond in a way that promotes healthier, more constructive relationships.

Exercise:

- Reflect on a recent interaction where emotions played a significant role. Did you respond with empathy and understanding? How could you have approached the situation differently? Practise acknowledging and validating the emotions of others in your next interaction.

Step 3: Surround Yourself with Positive Influences

The people you spend time with can significantly influence your mindset, behaviours, and outlook on life. Surrounding yourself with positive, supportive individuals helps reinforce your own positive habits and encourages personal growth. These are people who celebrate your successes, challenge you to be better, and offer encouragement when things get tough.

At the same time, it's important to recognise and distance yourself from individuals who drain your energy or engage in negative, toxic behaviours. Toxic relationships can lead to stress, self-doubt, and even hinder your progress. By curating your social circle, you can create an environment that fosters growth and positivity.

Exercise:

- Take stock of the people you spend the most time with. Are there individuals who leave you feeling energised and supported? Are there any relationships that are consistently draining or negative? Consider setting boundaries or reducing your time with those who have a negative impact.

Step 4: Seek Out Mentors and Role Models

Mentors and role models can provide invaluable guidance and support throughout your personal and professional journey. A mentor is someone who has experience in an area you wish to grow and is willing to share their knowledge, wisdom, and advice. Having a mentor offers you a safe space to ask questions, seek feedback, and receive encouragement.

Additionally, role models—people whose values and achievements inspire you—can offer motivation and perspective. Whether through books, talks, or personal connections, role models provide examples of what is possible and can guide you toward your own goals.

Exercise:

- Identify one person who could be a potential mentor in your life. Reach out to them with a request for advice or to explore how they could help you develop in your personal or professional life. Alternatively, find a role model whose journey you admire and use their story for inspiration.

Step 5: Offer Support to Others

Relationships are two-way streets. Just as you seek support from others, it's equally important to offer your support and encouragement to those around you. Being a supportive friend, colleague, or family member not only strengthens your connections but also fosters goodwill and trust.

Offering your time, listening ear, and advice when others need it can deepen relationships and create a sense of reciprocity. This mutual support network is an essential aspect of a thriving social circle. When you invest in others, you also create an environment where support is readily available when you need it.

Exercise:

- Think about someone in your life who may need your support. How can you offer help or encouragement? Consider reaching out to offer a kind word, lend a hand, or simply listen to their concerns.

Step 6: Develop Conflict Resolution Skills

Even in the best relationships, disagreements and misunderstandings can occur. The ability to navigate conflict with grace and understanding is an essential skill for maintaining healthy relationships. When conflicts arise, focus on resolving issues constructively rather than allowing them to escalate or fester.

Use "I" statements to express your feelings without blaming the other person, and be open to hearing their perspective. Compromise and collaboration are key to finding solutions that work for both parties. By addressing conflict with a calm, empathetic approach, you can strengthen relationships and build trust.

Exercise:

- Think about a past conflict in your life. How was it handled? Reflect on how you could have approached the situation with more understanding and empathy. Next time a conflict arises, practise addressing it in a calm and constructive manner.

Step 7: Make Time for Relationships

In our busy lives, it's easy to let relationships take a back seat. However, prioritising quality time with those you care about is essential for maintaining strong, supportive relationships. Whether it's scheduling regular catch-ups with friends, spending quality time with family, or connecting with colleagues, make an effort to invest in your relationships.

Small gestures, like a thoughtful message, a spontaneous phone call, or organising a regular catch-up, can go a long way in nurturing the bonds you share with others.

Exercise:

- Look at your calendar and set aside specific time slots for nurturing your key relationships. Whether it's a weekly call with a friend or a monthly dinner with family, commit to making these connections a priority.

Moving Forward with Stronger Relationships

Cultivating relationships and building a support system takes time and effort, but the rewards are immense. By investing in meaningful connections, setting boundaries, and offering support to others, you create an environment that promotes personal growth, emotional well-being, and success.

Remember that relationships are not only about receiving support but also about giving it. By fostering positive, reciprocal connections, you create a network that helps everyone thrive, including yourself.

Moving Forward with Purpose

Chapter 11: Staying Motivated and Overcoming Plateaus

Introduction

Motivation is the driving force behind every goal we set. It fuels our determination, pushes us through challenges, and helps us maintain focus on what we want to achieve. However, there will inevitably be times when our motivation wanes, and we find ourselves stuck in a plateau—those periods when progress feels slow or nonexistent. This chapter will explore strategies to help you stay motivated, push through plateaus, and maintain momentum on your journey toward achieving your goals.

Why Motivation Fades

Motivation is not a constant force. It ebbs and flows depending on various factors, such as our emotional state, external circumstances, and the challenges we face. At the start of a new goal, we often experience an initial burst of enthusiasm, but over time, this excitement can fade. As the novelty wears off and the reality of hard work sets in, it's easy to lose sight of our vision.

Plateaus often occur when we've made significant progress but feel as though we're no longer advancing. This can lead to frustration and self-doubt. However, understanding that plateaus are a normal part of the process can help you approach these moments with patience and resilience.

Step 1: Break Down Long-Term Goals into Smaller, Achievable Steps

One of the main reasons we lose motivation is that our goals seem too large or distant. When faced with a big, overwhelming task, it's easy to feel disheartened and question whether we'll ever reach our destination. To combat this, break your long-term goals down into smaller, more manageable tasks.

By setting smaller milestones, you give yourself regular opportunities to celebrate progress and stay motivated. These milestones act as checkpoints, allowing you to track your journey and recognise the achievements you've made. Each time you complete one of these smaller steps, you'll gain a sense of accomplishment and renew your motivation to continue moving forward.

Exercise:

- Take a large goal you're working towards and break it down into at least five smaller tasks or milestones. Set a timeline for each task and celebrate your progress as you complete each one.

Step 2: Revisit Your "Why"

When motivation starts to fade, it's important to reconnect with the reason you started in the first place. Your "why" is the deeper purpose or driving force behind your goal, and revisiting it can reignite your passion and determination. Ask yourself: Why is this goal important to me? What will achieving it mean for my life?

When you remind yourself of the emotional significance of your goal, it becomes easier to push through moments of doubt and stagnation. This deeper connection to your goal fuels your perseverance and helps you stay focused during tough times.

Exercise:

- Write down the reasons why your goal is important to you. How will it improve your life, your well-being, or your future? Keep this list somewhere visible as a reminder of your motivation.

Step 3: Create a Routine and Stick to It

One of the most effective ways to stay motivated is to create a consistent routine that incorporates actions toward your goal. Routines reduce the need for willpower, as they make progress feel automatic. The more ingrained your actions become, the less mental energy you need to stay motivated.

By scheduling time each day or week to focus on your goal, you build momentum that can carry you through challenging periods. Even on days when your motivation feels low, sticking to your routine ensures that you're making progress, no matter how small.

Exercise:

- Create a daily or weekly routine that includes specific actions towards your goal. Set aside time each day to work on one task, even if it's just for 15-20 minutes. Consistency is key.

Step 4: Embrace the Power of Accountability

Accountability can be a powerful motivator. When we have someone to answer to, whether it's a friend, mentor, or accountability partner, we're more likely to stay committed and take action. Knowing that someone else is tracking our progress can push us to show up, even when we don't feel like it.

You can set up accountability systems in many ways. For example, you might check in with someone regularly to share your progress, or you could track your goal publicly (e.g., on social media, in a blog, or with a group of like-minded individuals). Being accountable to someone else helps you stay on track, even when motivation is lacking.

Exercise:

- Find an accountability partner or group that shares similar goals or interests. Agree to check in with each other regularly to report your progress and offer support.

Step 5: Celebrate Small Wins and Progress

Motivation thrives on recognition and reward. It's easy to overlook small victories when we're focused on the bigger picture, but recognising your progress, no matter how minor, can reignite your enthusiasm. Take time to celebrate every milestone, as this positive reinforcement helps you stay motivated for the long haul.

Rewards don't have to be extravagant—simple gestures like treating yourself to something you enjoy, taking a break, or reflecting on how far you've come can provide the motivation needed to continue.

Exercise:

- After achieving a small milestone, celebrate! This could be through a small treat, a day off, or simply reflecting on your success. Recognise how far you've come to keep your motivation strong.

Step 6: Focus on the Process, Not Just the Outcome

During periods of stagnation, it's helpful to shift your focus from the end result to the process itself. Often, we become so fixated on the goal that we forget to enjoy the journey. Embrace the process of learning, improving, and growing, rather than just the outcome.

By focusing on the daily actions and progress you're making, you reduce the pressure of reaching the finish line and allow yourself to enjoy the experience. This shift in focus can help ease feelings of frustration and reignite your passion for the task at hand.

Exercise:

- Reflect on the process of achieving your goal. What have you learned along the way? What skills have you developed? Celebrate the progress you've made in developing new habits and strengths, regardless of the final outcome.

Step 7: Re-evaluate and Adjust Your Approach

Sometimes, plateaus occur because we've outgrown our current approach, or it's no longer working as effectively as it once did. When you feel stuck, it's worth taking a step back and evaluating your strategy. Are there any changes you can make to reinvigorate your progress? Is there a different method or approach that could yield better results?

Reassessing your plan and making adjustments can breathe new life into your goal, helping you get back on track and overcome the plateau.

Exercise:

- Take a moment to reflect on your progress and current approach. Are there any changes you can make to your strategy to help you move forward? Adjust your plan as needed and take action to get back on track.

Moving Forward with Motivation and Persistence

Motivation isn't something that always comes easily, especially during difficult or stagnant periods. However, by incorporating the strategies outlined in this chapter—such as breaking down goals, revisiting your "why," creating routines, and celebrating progress—you can stay motivated and keep pushing through plateaus.

Remember, plateaus are a natural part of the journey, and they don't mean you've failed. They're simply moments for reflection and growth. By staying persistent and flexible, you can continue making progress and move closer to achieving your goals.

Chapter 12: Reflect, Refine, and Progress

Introduction

The pursuit of any goal requires consistent effort, but it also demands reflection and adjustment. It's easy to get caught up in the hustle of day-to-day tasks, pushing forward without taking the time to assess our progress or consider what changes may be necessary. In this chapter, we'll explore the importance of reflection in your journey, how to refine your approach based on what you've learned, and how to keep moving forward with purpose and intention.

Why Reflection is Essential

Reflection is a powerful tool that allows us to pause, step back, and gain perspective on our progress. It helps us understand what's working, what isn't, and what adjustments might be needed. Without reflection, it's easy to repeat the same mistakes, stay stuck in unproductive habits, or miss opportunities for improvement.

By regularly taking time to reflect, you gain clarity about your goals and can refine your approach, ensuring that your actions remain aligned with your long-term vision. Reflection helps you grow not just in terms of achievements, but in understanding your motivations, strengths, and areas for development.

Step 1: Set Aside Time for Regular Reflection

To truly benefit from reflection, you need to make it a habit. Set aside time regularly—whether weekly, monthly, or quarterly—to look back on your progress and assess where you are in relation to your goals. This can be as simple as taking a few minutes at the end of each day to reflect, or a more structured approach, such as a monthly review of your accomplishments and challenges.

During these sessions, ask yourself questions such as:

- What progress have I made since my last reflection?
- What obstacles have I encountered, and how did I handle them?
- What have I learned about myself during this process?
- Are my goals still aligned with my values and priorities?

Exercise:

- Set aside 30 minutes at the end of each week to reflect on your progress. Use the questions above to guide your reflection and make notes on any adjustments you may need to make moving forward.

Step 2: Learn from Your Setbacks

Setbacks are an inevitable part of any journey, and it's how we respond to them that determines our success. Instead of viewing setbacks as failures, see them as learning opportunities. Reflect on what went wrong, what could have been done differently, and what lessons you can take forward.

Embrace the mindset that each setback is a chance to refine your approach, become more resilient, and grow stronger. The key is to not get discouraged by mistakes but to use them as stepping stones toward greater success. Remember, growth isn't linear, and setbacks are often where the most valuable lessons are learned.

Exercise:

- Think about a recent setback or challenge you faced. Write down what you learned from it and how you plan to approach similar situations in the future. What can you do differently next time to ensure greater success?

Step 3: Refine Your Strategy Based on Insights

Once you've reflected on your progress and learned from any setbacks, it's time to refine your strategy. It's essential to recognise that your original plan may not always be the best route to success. As you gain new insights, refine your approach to make it more effective.

Ask yourself:

- Are the methods I'm using still serving me well?
- Are there any new skills or knowledge I've gained that I should apply?
- Is there a more efficient or productive way to achieve my goals?

Adapting your strategy doesn't mean abandoning your goals; it means being flexible and open to adjusting your approach to achieve better results. This continuous process of refinement ensures that your path remains aligned with your evolving needs and circumstances.

Exercise:

- Review your current approach to a specific goal. Identify one area where you could refine your strategy to make your progress more efficient or effective. Implement this change in the coming week and assess its impact.

Step 4: Maintain Momentum by Setting New Challenges

Even after you've made progress and refined your strategy, it's important to maintain momentum by setting new challenges. Stagnation occurs when we stop growing or challenging ourselves. Once you've achieved a goal, take time to celebrate your success, but don't let it be the end of your journey.

Set new challenges that stretch your capabilities and encourage further growth. These challenges could be related to your current goal or something entirely new, depending on where you are in your journey. The key is to keep evolving and setting new benchmarks that push you to become the best version of yourself.

Exercise:

- Think about the next step after reaching your current goal. What new challenge can you set for yourself? This might be a more advanced version of your original goal or something entirely different that excites and motivates you.

Step 5: Cultivate a Habit of Continuous Learning

One of the most effective ways to keep progressing is to cultivate a mindset of continuous learning. In today's fast-paced world, there is always more to learn, whether it's about your goals, your field of work, or yourself. The most successful people are those who are committed to lifelong learning, constantly seeking ways to improve and grow.

To support your personal growth, make learning a regular part of your routine. This might involve reading books, taking courses, attending workshops, or seeking advice from mentors. By dedicating time to expand your knowledge and skills, you'll ensure that your personal development doesn't plateau.

Exercise:

- Choose one area of your life or goal that you'd like to learn more about. Find a book, course, or resource that will help deepen your knowledge. Set a goal to engage with it for at least 30 minutes each week.

Step 6: Celebrate Your Achievements

As you reflect, refine, and progress, it's crucial to take the time to celebrate your achievements, no matter how small. Celebrating your successes reinforces positive behaviour, boosts morale, and motivates you to keep going. It also gives you an opportunity to appreciate the effort you've put in and acknowledge how far you've come.

Celebrating doesn't always have to involve grand gestures; simple actions like taking a moment to acknowledge your progress, treating yourself to something small, or sharing your success with others can be just as powerful.

Exercise:

- Reflect on a recent achievement, whether it's a milestone or a completed task. Take a moment to celebrate this success, whether by treating yourself, sharing the accomplishment with a friend, or simply taking a moment of gratitude.

Moving Forward with Clarity and Purpose

The process of reflecting, refining, and progressing is an ongoing journey that allows you to stay aligned with your goals, learn from your experiences, and continue growing. By regularly assessing your progress, making adjustments, and setting new challenges, you ensure that you're always moving forward with intention and purpose.

Remember, growth is not about reaching a final destination but about continuously evolving. By embracing reflection and adaptation, you create a cycle of progress that leads to ongoing personal development and success.

Chapter 13: Setting Goals and Taking Consistent Action

Introduction

Goals are the compass that guide us towards the life we desire. Without clear goals, it's easy to drift aimlessly, reacting to the demands of life without a sense of direction or purpose. In this chapter, we'll explore how to set effective goals that align with your values, and how to take consistent action to achieve them. The key to success is not just having goals, but staying focused and committed to them, even when faced with challenges.

Why Setting Goals is Crucial

Goals give us direction and purpose. They provide a clear vision of where we want to go and act as a blueprint for getting there. Without goals, we might feel overwhelmed by the tasks in front of us, unsure of what to prioritise. By setting goals, we create a roadmap that helps us focus our energy, time, and resources on what truly matters.

Additionally, goals help measure progress. They allow us to track our achievements, reassess when needed, and make adjustments to stay on course. Without goals, it's easy to feel like you're busy but not actually making meaningful progress.

Step 1: Define Your Goals Clearly

The first step to achieving any goal is to define it clearly. A vague goal is difficult to act on, so make sure your goal is specific, measurable, and time-bound. Use the SMART framework to ensure your goals are clear and actionable:

- **Specific**: What exactly do you want to achieve?
- **Measurable**: How will you track progress and know when the goal is achieved?

- **Achievable**: Is this goal realistic and within your capacity?
- **Relevant**: Does it align with your broader life values and long-term aspirations?
- **Time-bound**: What is your deadline for achieving this goal?

For example, instead of setting a vague goal like "I want to get fit," a SMART goal would be "I want to run 5 km in under 30 minutes within the next three months."

Exercise:

- Take a goal you're currently working on and refine it using the SMART framework. Write down your goal with specific details, a timeline, and how you will measure your progress.

Step 2: Break Goals into Smaller Steps

A large goal can often feel overwhelming. Breaking it down into smaller, more manageable steps makes it easier to focus on the next immediate task, rather than becoming discouraged by the scale of the entire goal. These smaller steps act as checkpoints, and completing each one builds momentum and confidence.

For example, if your goal is to launch a business, break it down into smaller steps such as:

1. Researching your market and competitors
2. Writing a business plan
3. Securing funding
4. Setting up your website and brand
5. Marketing your product

By breaking the larger goal into smaller, more achievable tasks, you make progress feel more tangible and less intimidating.

Exercise:

- Take one of your larger goals and break it down into smaller, specific actions. Set deadlines for each step and begin focusing on completing them one at a time.

Step 3: Create a Consistent Action Plan

Once you've broken your goals down into smaller tasks, it's time to create a plan for how you will consistently take action. This is where the key to success lies—consistency. It's easy to get excited about a goal in the beginning, but it's the daily actions you take that lead to success.

Make time each day or week to work on your goal. Whether it's 15 minutes of writing, a 30-minute workout, or 1 hour of studying, the most important thing is to make it a regular habit. Consistent action, even in small amounts, builds momentum and brings you closer to your desired outcome.

Exercise:

- Create a weekly schedule that includes specific time blocks for working on your goal. Make these time blocks non-negotiable—treat them like appointments that can't be missed.

Step 4: Stay Accountable

Accountability is a powerful motivator. When we know that someone else is expecting us to follow through on our commitments, we're more likely to stay focused and consistent. Find an accountability partner, whether it's a friend, family member, or mentor, who can check in with you and offer support.

Alternatively, you can use digital tools like habit trackers or project management apps to monitor your progress. Tracking your own progress helps you stay motivated and gives you a sense of accomplishment as you check off each completed task.

Exercise:

- Find an accountability partner to help you stay on track. Agree on how often you'll check in with each other and what kind of support you'll offer.

Step 5: Adjust and Refine as You Go

It's important to remain flexible as you work towards your goals. The path to success is rarely a straight line, and obstacles may arise that cause you to adjust your plans. Be open to change and refine your approach as needed.

If you find that one method isn't working, experiment with another approach. If you're not making progress as quickly as you'd like, reassess your timeline and set new milestones. The most successful people aren't those who never face challenges, but those who keep adjusting and moving forward, no matter the setbacks.

Exercise:

- Reflect on any areas of your current goals where you might need to adjust your approach. Are there new resources or techniques you can try to make progress? Set new targets if necessary and adapt your plan to ensure continued success.

Step 6: Celebrate Milestones and Keep Pushing Forward

Taking time to celebrate small wins is essential for maintaining motivation. Each time you reach a milestone, reward yourself. These celebrations don't need to be extravagant, but recognising your achievements along the way keeps you motivated and reinforces the positive behaviour.

However, celebration doesn't mean stopping. Use each milestone as a reminder that you're capable of achieving your larger goal. Acknowledge your progress, but keep your eyes on the next task. Maintaining momentum means recognising your success while always looking forward to the next step.

Exercise:

- Identify one recent milestone in your journey toward your goal. Celebrate this achievement by treating yourself to something small that brings you joy.

Step 7: Maintain a Growth Mindset

Finally, it's essential to maintain a growth mindset throughout your journey. A growth mindset is the belief that your abilities can be developed through effort, learning, and persistence. When faced with challenges or setbacks, view them as opportunities for growth and learning.

Instead of thinking, "I can't do this," say, "I can't do this yet." By maintaining a growth mindset, you stay open to learning, improving, and adjusting your approach to achieve success.

Exercise:

- Reflect on a recent challenge or setback you've faced. How did you respond? Next time you face a similar obstacle, remind yourself to embrace it as an opportunity to learn and grow.

Moving Forward with Purpose and Determination

Setting goals and taking consistent action is the foundation for success. It requires clarity, discipline, and persistence, but with the right mindset and approach, you can achieve anything you set your mind to. By following the steps outlined in this chapter—defining clear goals, breaking them down into manageable steps, creating a consistent plan, staying accountable, and maintaining a growth mindset—you'll be well on your way to turning your dreams into reality.

Real Life Examples

Chapter 1: Identifying Your Goals

J.K. Rowling and Writing "Harry Potter" When J.K. Rowling set out to write the *Harry Potter* series, she had a clear vision of creating a world where readers could escape and experience the magic of books. Her initial goal was not just to write a story, but to create a lasting impact on children's literature. Her first book was rejected by multiple publishers before it was finally accepted. The process was long and challenging, but Rowling's clear vision and goal—creating a book that would captivate readers—kept her going.

Note: Setting a clear, meaningful goal allows you to keep moving forward, even when faced with rejection or setbacks.

Chapter 2: Understanding Limiting Beliefs

Michael Jordan and Overcoming Self-Doubt Michael Jordan, often considered the greatest basketball player of all time, was famously cut from his high school basketball team. This could have led to a limiting belief that he wasn't good enough, but instead, Jordan used this setback as motivation. He worked tirelessly on his skills and developed a mindset that allowed him to push past his doubts and limitations.

Note: Rather than being defined by a setback, use it as fuel to challenge limiting beliefs and work towards success.

Chapter 3: Developing a Growth Mindset

Thomas Edison and the Light Bulb Thomas Edison is known for inventing the electric light bulb, but what is less well-known is that he faced countless failures before achieving success. In fact, when asked about his numerous unsuccessful attempts, Edison famously said, "I have not failed. I've just found 10,000 ways that won't work." Edison's growth mindset allowed him to view each failure as a step toward success rather than a reason to give up.

Note: A growth mindset helps you embrace failure as part of the learning process, ultimately leading to success.

Chapter 4: Building Confidence Through Action

Example: Oprah Winfrey's Journey to Confidence Oprah Winfrey faced a difficult start in life, including abuse and poverty, but she overcame these challenges and built her confidence over time. As she worked her way up in media, she often faced rejection and doubt. However, through consistent action—such as honing her interview skills, building relationships, and expanding her platform—Oprah became a trusted and influential figure in media.

Note: Confidence is built through consistent action. The more you practise and refine your skills, the more confident you become.

Chapter 5: Time Management and Prioritisation

Elon Musk and Time Blocking Elon Musk is known for managing multiple companies simultaneously, including Tesla and SpaceX. He uses a time-blocking method to manage his incredibly busy schedule. Musk divides his day into five-minute blocks, ensuring he remains focused and productive, even with a packed agenda. This strategy allows him to prioritise his most important tasks and maintain productivity across his ventures.

Note: Effective time management, such as time-blocking, can help you focus on what truly matters and maximise your productivity.

Chapter 6: Building Positive Habits

James Clear and Habit Formation James Clear, the author of *Atomic Habits*, spent years experimenting with habits to improve his life. One example he shares is the simple act of going to the gym. By making it a non-negotiable daily habit, he was able to build consistency, which later became a cornerstone of his personal and professional life. Clear emphasises that small, incremental improvements compound over time, leading to massive results.

Note: Small, consistent actions lead to significant long-term results when they become habits.

Chapter 7: Practising Self-Care and Mental Well-being

Arianna Huffington and the Importance of Sleep Arianna Huffington, the founder of *The Huffington Post*, experienced burnout after pushing herself too hard in her career. After collapsing from exhaustion, she recognised the importance of self-care, particularly sleep. She made sleep a priority and wrote *The Sleep Revolution* to raise awareness about its importance. Today, she advocates for balance and well-being, prioritising rest as essential for peak performance.

Note: Prioritising self-care and mental well-being is crucial for long-term success. Without proper rest and recovery, even the most ambitious goals can suffer.

Chapter 8: Cultivating Relationships and Support Systems

Steve Jobs and the Role of Mentorship Steve Jobs, the co-founder of Apple, had an important mentor in his life—Mike Markkula, an early investor in Apple. Markkula's guidance helped Jobs navigate the challenges of building Apple into one of the most successful companies in the world. In return, Jobs mentored others, including his team at Apple, creating a network of support that helped drive innovation and growth.

Note: Cultivating strong relationships and seeking mentorship helps provide guidance, accountability, and support in achieving your goals.

Chapter 9: Staying Motivated and Overcoming Plateaus

Williams and Perseverance Serena Williams has faced numerous setbacks throughout her career, including injuries and personal challenges. Despite these obstacles, she has continued to come back stronger each time. After a lengthy injury hiatus, Williams returned to the court with determination and won several Grand Slam titles, defying expectations and overcoming plateaus.

Note: Even when progress slows down or plateaus, perseverance and maintaining a positive mindset can help you push through and continue achieving.

Chapter 10: Reflect, Refine, and Progress

Warren Buffett's Approach to Reflecting and Refining Warren Buffett, one of the world's most successful investors, is known for regularly reflecting on his investment strategies. He spends a significant portion of his day reading and learning from both his successes and mistakes. This process of reflection allows him to refine his approach and continue making informed, thoughtful decisions in his investments.

Note: Regular reflection is essential for growth. By taking time to reassess and refine your strategy, you ensure continuous progress toward your goals.

Chapter 11: Setting Goals and Taking Consistent Action

Richard Branson and Goal-Oriented Action Richard Branson, the founder of Virgin Group, set an ambitious goal at a young age to create a business empire. Through consistent action, Branson built a variety of successful companies, including Virgin Records and Virgin Atlantic. His ability to set clear goals, take bold action, and remain committed to his vision allowed him to overcome the many challenges that came with entrepreneurship.

Note: Setting clear, actionable goals and consistently working towards them, even in the face of adversity, is key to long-term success.

Conclusion

These real-life examples demonstrate the power of setting clear goals, taking consistent action, and maintaining a growth mindset. Whether facing setbacks or building on success, each person's journey is marked by perseverance, reflection, and a willingness to learn and adapt. By incorporating these lessons into your own life, you can overcome obstacles, stay motivated, and achieve your personal and professional goals.